Complete Guide for your Nuwave Oven

Top 50 Nuwave Recipes to Make your Life Easier and Tastier

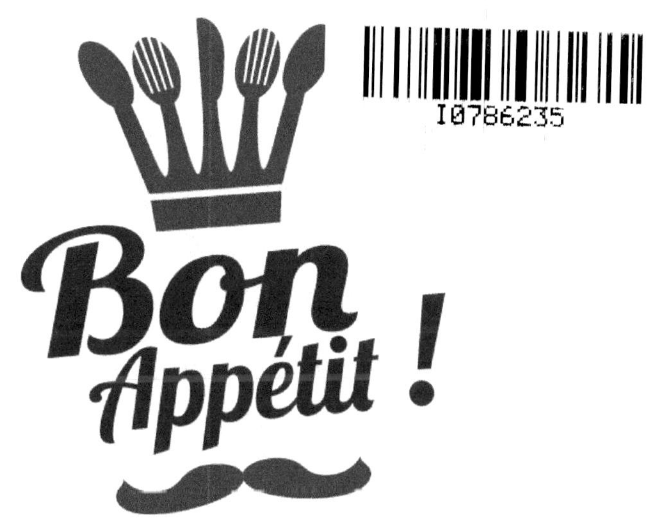

Judy Preston

Text Copyright © Judy Preston

Legal & Disclaimer

to your doctor, attorney, financial advisor or such other professional advisor) before using any of the suggested remedies, techniques, or information in this book.

Upon using the contents and information contained in this book, you agree to hold harmless the Author from and against any damages, costs, and expenses, including any legal fees potentially resulting from the application of any of the information provided by this book. This disclaimer applies to any loss, damages or injury caused by the use and application, whether directly or indirectly, of any advice or information presented, whether for breach of contract, tort, negligence, personal injury, criminal intent, or under any other cause of action.

You agree to accept all risks of using the information presented inside this book.

You agree that by continuing to read this book, where appropriate and/or necessary, you shall consult a professional (including but not limited to your doctor, attorney, or financial advisor or such other advisor as needed) before using any of the suggested remedies, techniques, or information in this book.

Table of Contents

Introduction

If you have a NuWave oven and you don't know how to use it effectively, nuwave oven recipes will Guide to a Fast and sure Way of Cooking different recipes.

This cookbook has the information required to know about your NuWave Oven. It has the guide on how to operate it, the advantages of its usage, the temperature conversion guide, and the delightful recipes that are very swift to prepare using the NuWave Oven. These recipes have been arranged into five different groupings for the ease of all the users.

The NuWave Oven is known for its ultraviolet heat in cooking healthy food faster and efficient than other conventional ovens. It will help you save time whether you're cooking, roasting, broiling, grilling, baking, steaming, or air-frying using less energy.

The NuWave Oven is very swift in usage. The default temperature is 350 degrees Fahrenheit which is adjustable depending on the meals you are making. The range of the temperature is 100 - 350 degrees Fahrenheit. If you set the temp, you will also have to adjust the cooking time as well. And if you doubt if the food is as delicious as what you anticipated, you'll just have to press the pause or clear button to check and hit the start button to continue. If you want to resume on your cooking time, you just double press the pause button.

Cooking with the Nuwave Oven has several advantages

 Great Technology advancement as it has the triple combo power that differentiates it from other ovens.

The heat is conducted directly.

The nuwave oven uses a fan to circulate hot are around your meal

It cooks your food perfectly.

This oven produces healthy meals as it extracts all excess fat from the food by its fat dripping cooking style while the food remains tasty and tender on the inside.

The nuwave oven is portable due to its lighter weight compared to other ovens. It is therefore easy to carry along.

It is easy to clean as all the parts of nuwave oven can be dipped in the dishwasher apart from the power head.

Breakfast Recipes

Nuwave Oven Bacon

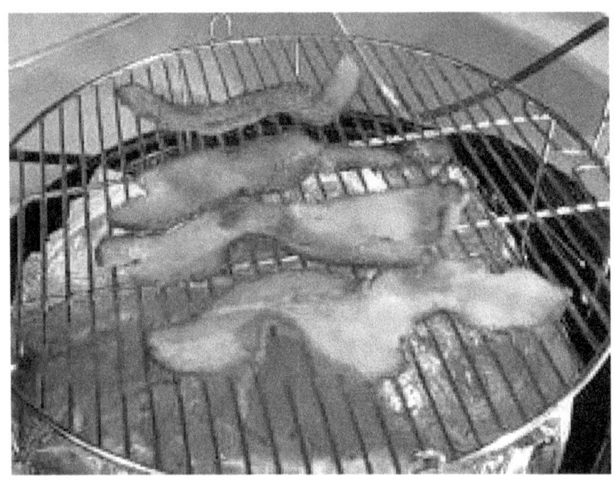

Prep time: 5 mins

Servings: 6

Ingredients:

- 12 slices bacon

Preparation:

1. Line bottom of the oven with foil to catch bacon grease.

2. Place bacon slices on 4-inch rack.

3. Cook on High power (350 degrees F) for 8 minutes. Turn the bacon over and cook for an

extra 5 mins or till the bacon reaches desired crispness.

4. Serve straightaway.

5. Enjoy!

Nutritional Info:

Calories: 541

Total Fat: 42g

Total carbs: 1.4g

Protein: 37 g

Ham, Cheese, and Bacon Quiche

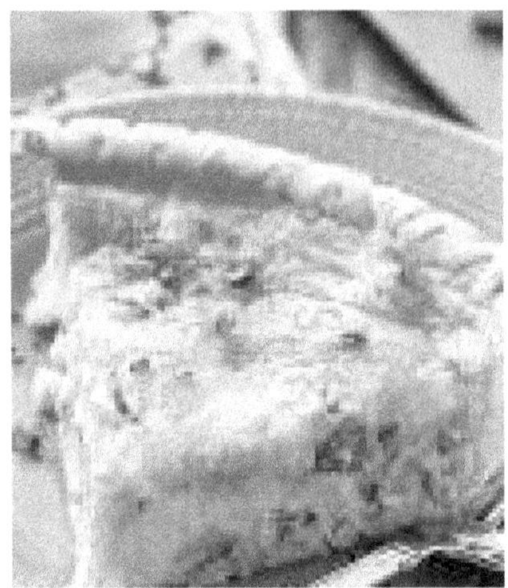

Prep time: 10 mins

Servings: 8

Ingredients:

- Pie crust

- 1 c. ham, diced

- 4 bacon slices

- 1 ½ c. shredded cheddar cheese

- 1 tbsp. flour

- 3 large eggs

- 1½ c. milk

- Sea salt

- Black pepper

Preparation:

1. Place pie crust on the 1-inch rack and bake on High power (350 degrees) for 6-7 mins, till it starts to brown. Remove from oven for cooling.

2. Spread ham and bacon uniformly across the bottommost of pie crust. Dust cheese evenly on top.

3. In a large bowl, mix flour, large eggs, milk, salt, and pepper then pour the mixture into the pie crust.

4. Place on 1-inch rack and bake on High power 350°C for 15 mins. Decrease heat to Power Level 8 (300 degrees F) and cook for an additional 10 mins or until a toothpick inserted in centre comes out clear. Let quiche sit for 10 mins before slicing. Serve warm.

Nutritional Info:

Calories: 220.0

Total Fat: 7.2g

Total carbs: 22.6g

Protein: 15.3g

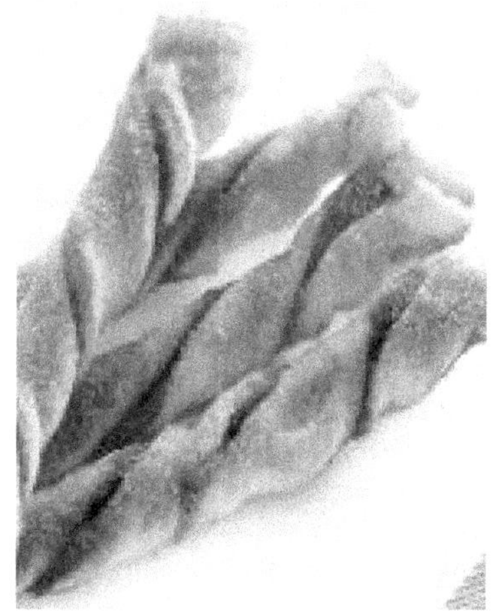

Prep time: 5 mins

Servings: 3

Ingredients:

- 1 tsp. cinnamon

- ½ c. brown sugar

- 11 oz. frozen breadsticks

Preparation:

1. Mix the cinnamon and brown sugar in a medium-sized bowl. Whisk together by a wire whisk till it is combined. Put aside.

2. Pour the mixture into a flat plate.

3. Place a single breadstick in the cinnamon sugar mixture and roll until well coated.

4. Hold the breadstick from both ends in each hand and twist until you get a rope like texture.

5. Place on a 3-inch rack and bake on 'HI' for about 12 to 14 minutes, flipping it over at the halfway mark.

6. Serve immediately.

7. Enjoy!

Nutritional Info:

Calories: 170

Total Fat: 7g

Carbs: 26g

Protein: 1g

Healthy Low-Fat Granola

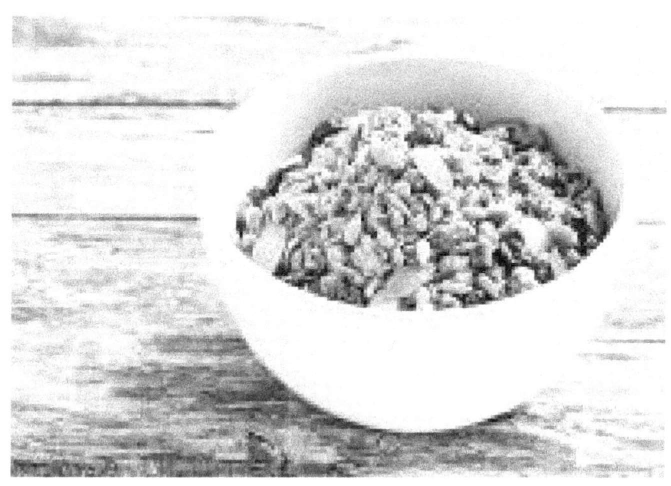

Prep time: 15 mins

Servings: 8

Ingredients:

- 4 c. old-fashioned oats
- ¼ c. flax seed
- ¼ c. wheat germ
- ¼ c. coconut flakes
- ¼ c. pumpkin or sunflower seeds
- ¼ c. sliced almonds
- 1/3 c. maple syrup

- ¼ c apple juice

- Cinnamon

- Vanilla

- Salt

Preparation:

1. Mix all the ingredients in a large bowl. Stir thoroughly in order to coat all ingredients.

2. Line rimmed cooking sheet with parchment paper. Spread mixture uniformly on cooking sheet.

3. Place pan in NuWave on 1-inch rack. Cook at 350 degrees at a power level high for 10 minutes. Stir, and cook for an addition 10-15 minutes, until lightly browned.

Nutritional Info:

Calories: 381.2

Total Fat: 5.6g

Carbs: 79.3g

Protein: 8.5g

Cheese Frittata with Basil

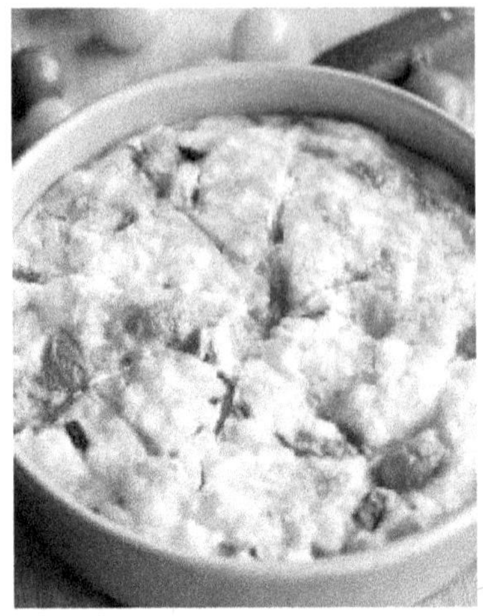

Prep time: 15minutes

Servings: 4 cheese frittata

Ingredients:

- 1 tbsp. virgin olive oil

- 1 chopped yellow onion

- 8 eggs

- ½ c. milk

- ½ tsp. salt

- ¼ tsp. ground pepper

- 6 oz. chopped tomatoes

- ½ c. goat cheese

- ½ c. basil, chopped

Preparation:

1. Heat the virgin olive oil in a pan over standard heat and fry the onions until translucent, 3-4 minutes.

2. Whisk together eggs and milk in a large bowl. Add salt and pepper seasonings. Fold in sun-dried tomatoes, goat cheese, and basil, and onion.

3. Pour egg mixture into the pan. Bake on High power (350 degrees F) for 36 to 40 mins, or till toothpick in centre comes out clear. If the top becomes too brown, cover with foil during last stage of cooking.

4. Serve frittata immediately or allow to cool to room temperature. May also be refrigerated for up to 1 day and served cold.

Nutritional Info:

Calories: 146

Fats: 8g

Protein: 9g

Carbs: 11g

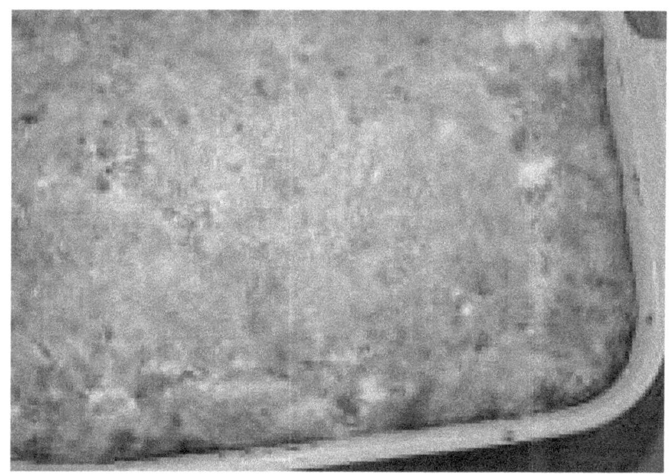

Prep time: 5 mins

Servings: 2

Ingredients:

- 5 eggs
- 3 oz. shredded Cheddar cheese
- ¼ c. milk
- ½ c. bacon or ham
- 1/8 c. chopped onion
- ¼ c. chopped green pepper
- ½ tbsp. parsley

Preparation:

1. Put the eggs in a medium-sized mixing bowl and add in the milk then beat using a whisk until the eggs get a fluffy texture.

2. Add the cheese, green pepper, bacon or ham and onion and mix well.

3. Pour the egg and meat mixture in a 4-inch by 4-inch silicon baking dish (grease if you are using a normal baking rack).

4. Put the baking dish on the 1-inch rack. Set temperature on the 'HI' setting and bake for about 10 to 15 minutes.

5. Let the egg sit in the in the dome with the heat off for another minute.

6. Extract the egg from the silicon-baking dish and slice into pieces.

7. Serve hot with a side dish of baked English muffins or whole wheat bread.

8. Enjoy!

Nutritional Info:

Calories: 194.0

Total Fat: 6.9g

Total carbs: 8.3g

Protein: 21.7g

Egg and Bacon Muffins

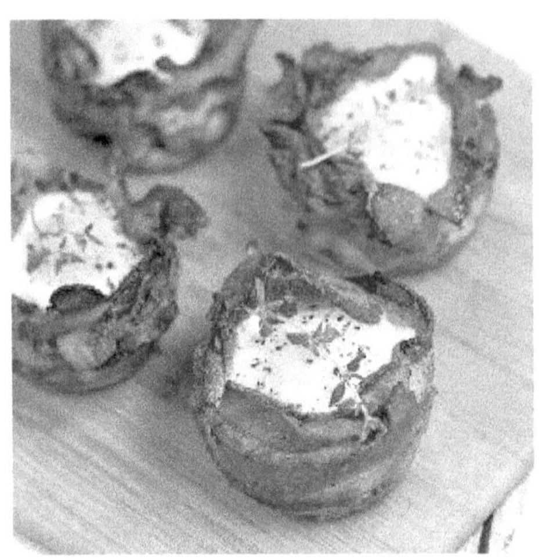

Prep time: 10 mins

Servings: 6

Ingredients:

- 5 eggs

- ½ c. bacon crumbles

- ¼ c. onion, chopped

- ¼ c. red bell pepper, chopped

- 4 tbsps. milk

- Sea salt

- Black pepper

- ¼ shredded cheddar cheese

Preparation:

1. Spray 6 cup muffin pot with culinary spray.

2. Beats eggs in big bowl. Stir in bacon crumbles, onion, bell pepper, salt, and pepper. Fold in grated cheese.

3. Spoon mixture into muffin cups.

4. Place muffin pan on 1-inch rack. Cook on High Power (350 degrees F) within 15-20 mins, till knife inserted in centre of a muffin comes out clear.

5. Serve warm.

6. Enjoy!

Nutritional Info:

Calories: 111.0

Total Fat: 8.1g

Total carbs: 0.6g

Protein: 8.2g

English muffin and Egg Casserole

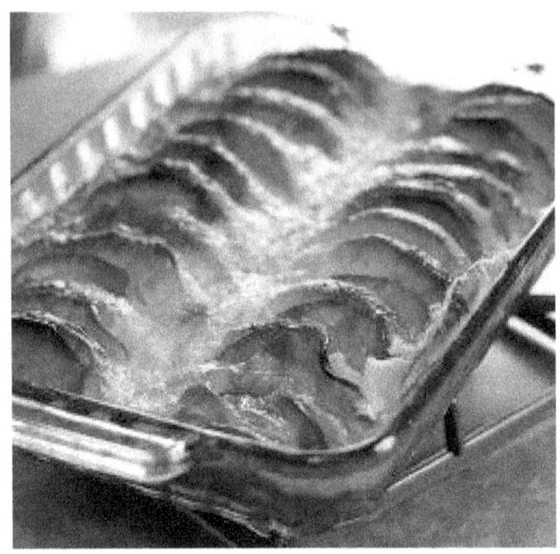

Prep time: 15 mins

Servings: 3 – 4

Ingredients:

- 12oz. muffins

- 3 eggs

- 3 slices chopped Canadian bacon

- ¾ c. milk

- 2 tsps. lemon juice

- 1 tbsp. mayonnaise

- 1 tsp. fresh lemon zest

- Butter

Preparation:

1. Cut the English muffins into two halves and then chop into 1-inch cubes.

2. Crack the eggs in a big mixing bowl and pour in milk. Whisk till fluffy.

3. Add chopped Canadian bacon, mayonnaise, fresh lemon juice, and fresh lemon zest to it and mix well until combined.

4. Add the English muffin cubes into the egg mixture and mix till fully coated.

5. Spray a 4-inch by 4-inch baking dish with cooking spray or grease it with butter.

6. Pour the prepared egg combination to the prepped baking rack then cover with an aluminium foil. Refrigerate for 6 to 8 hours or overnight.

7. Remove the aluminium foil and set it aside.

8. Place the uncovered baking dish on the 1inch rack.

9. Bake on the 'HI' setting for about 45 to 50 minutes.

10.   Cover using the reserved aluminium foil and continue baking for another 15-20 mins.

11.   Serve. Enjoy!

Nutritional Info:

Calories: 367.3

Total Fat: 14.6g

Total carbs: 44.5g

Protein: 14.7g

Crab Quiche

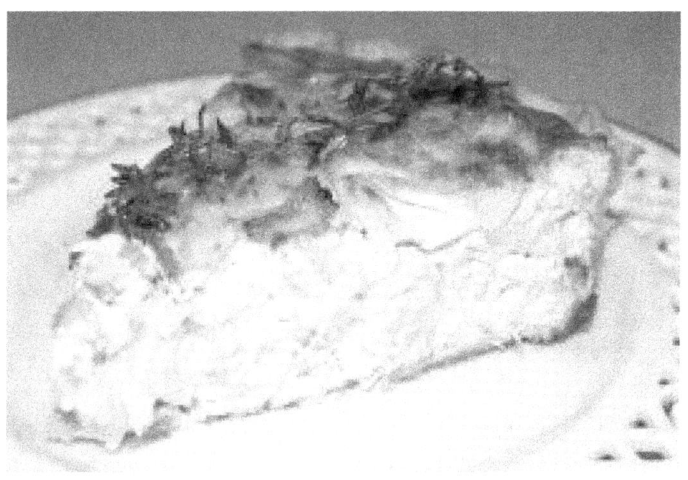

Prep time: 5 mins

Servings: 8

Ingredients:

- Pie crust

- 4 medium eggs

- 1 c. heavy cream

- ¼ tsp. Sea salt

- ¼ tsp. Black pepper

- 1tsp. hot sauce

- 1 c. Monterey Jack cheese, shredded

- ¼ c. Parmesan cheese, grated

- 1 chopped onion

- 2 cans lump crabmeat

Preparation:

1. Place pie crust on the 1-inch rack and bake on High power (350 degrees) for 6-7 mins or till it starts to brown. Remove from oven and allow cooling.

2. In a medium bowl, mix eggs, cream, salt, pepper, and hot sauce. Stir in cheeses, onion, and crabmeat.

3. Pour into pie crust.

4. Place on 1-inch rack and bake on power level High (350 °C) for 15 mins.

5. Reduce heat to Power level 8 (300 degrees F) and cook for an additional 10-15 mins or until a toothpick inserted in centre comes out clear. Allow to relax for 10 minutes before serving.

6. Enjoy!

Nutritional Info:

Calories: 148.0

Total Fat: 5.6g

Total carbs: 14.3g

Protein: 10.3g

Baked Eggs with Spinach and Tomatoes

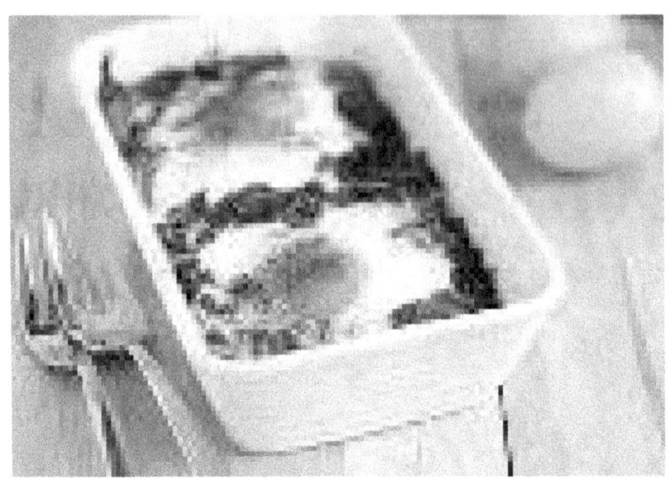

Prep time: 10 mins

Servings: 4

Ingredients:

- 8 oz. chopped spinach

- 3 chopped plum tomatoes

- ¼ tsp. garlic powder

- ¼ tsp. red pepper flakes

- Sea salt

- Black pepper

- 8 large eggs

- 2 tbsps. cream

- ½ c. shredded cheddar cheese

Preparation:

1. Spray casserole dish with cooking spray.

2. Squeeze out excess moisture from thawed spinach.

3. Spread tomatoes on the bottom of casserole dish. Layer spinach on top of tomatoes. Season with garlic powder, red pepper flakes, salt, and pepper. Crack eggs on top, drizzle with cream, and sprinkle with cheese.

4. Place dish on 1-inch rack. Bake on High power (350 °C) for 15 minutes or until egg whites are opaque.

5. Serve Immediately.

6. Enjoy!

Nutritional Info:

Calories: 114

Fat: 7g

Carbs: 3g

Protein: 9g

Meat Recipes

Lamb Meatballs

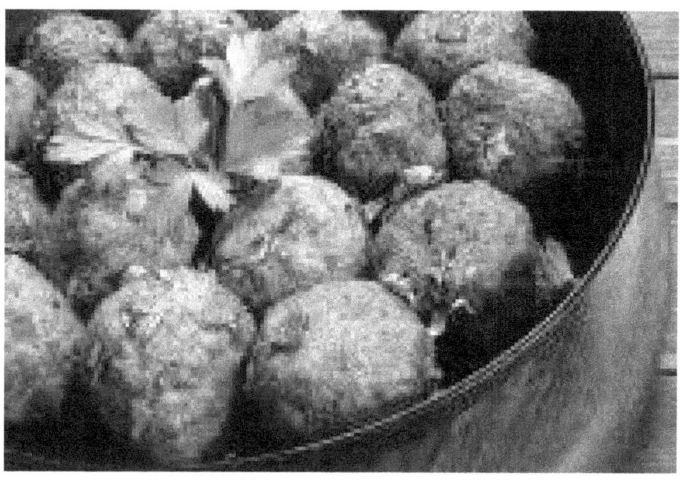

Prep time: 15 mins

Servings: 3

Ingredients:

- ½ lb. ground lamb

- ¼ tsp. cinnamon

- 2 tbsps. chopped scallions

- ½ tsp. ground cumin

- ½ tsp. salt

- ½ tsp. allspice

- 1 beaten egg

- 1 ½ tbsps. semolina

- 1 tbsp. chopped parsley.

Preparation:

1. Place the ground lamb and scallions in a large mixing bowl. Mix till well combined.

2. Add cinnamon, allspice, semolina, cumin and salt to the meat and scallion mix.

3. Pour the beaten egg over the spice-covered meat and use your hands to lightly knead until you get a semi-solid mix. Keep a bowl of cold water handy and constantly wet your palms. This will ensure that the meat doesn't get too sticky to work with.

4. Cover the bowl with a plastic wrap and refrigerate for about an 1 hour or until the meat is firm enough to retain its shape.

5. Divide the meat mixture into 3 parts (about 3 ounces each).

6. Apply oil on your palms and mould each meat portion into a round meatball.

7. Put the meatballs on a 3-inch rack and grill on the 'HI' setting for about 20 to 25 minutes. Pause the oven around the 12-minute mark and turn the meatballs over.

8. Once the meatballs are done, serve hot over a bed of pasta, topped with the sauce of your choice.

9. Enjoy!

Nutritional Info:

Calories: 93.0

Total Fat: 5.9g

Total carbs: 4.8g

Protein: 5.0g

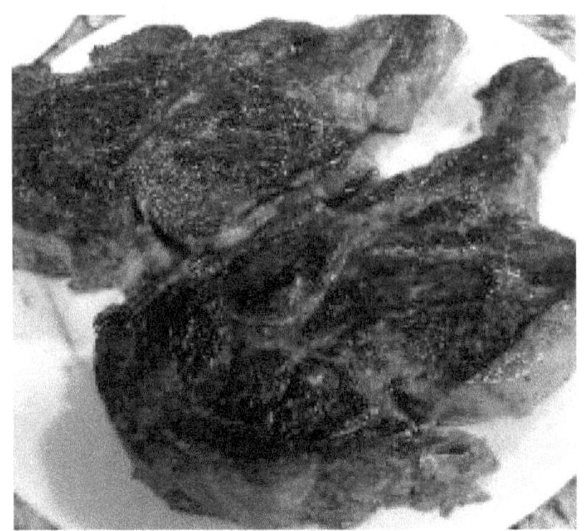

Prep time: 15 mins

Servings: 4

Ingredients:

- Fresh ginger

- ¼ c. sesame oil

- 8 minced garlic cloves

- 2 tsps. lemon juice

- 1 tbsp. honey

- 1 tsps. salt

- 1 tsp. ground pepper

- 1½ lbs. trimmed flank steak

Preparation:

1. In a medium bowl, whisk all ingredients except steak. Pour into the large resealable plastic bag.

2. Add flank steak, seal, and shake thoroughly to the coat steak with marinade.

3. Allow to marinade for 30 mins at room temperature. Can also marinate in the refrigerator for up to 24 hours.

4. Remove steak from marinade, allow excess marinade to drip off. Ensure liner is at the base of oven and place steak on the 4-inch rack. Cook steaks on High power until desired doneness, flipping once during cooking. For rare, cook 5-6 minutes per side; for medium rare, cook 6-7 mins each side; for medium, cook 7-8 mins each side, and for well-done cook 9-10 minutes each side. Insert meat thermometer to check for doneness.

5. Remove from oven and place on chopping board and let rest for 5-10 minutes. Slice, against the grain to thin slices. Serve.

Nutritional Info:

Calories: 215.0

Total Fat: 11.8g

Total carbs: 2.9g

Protein: 23.5g

Yankee Style Pot Roast

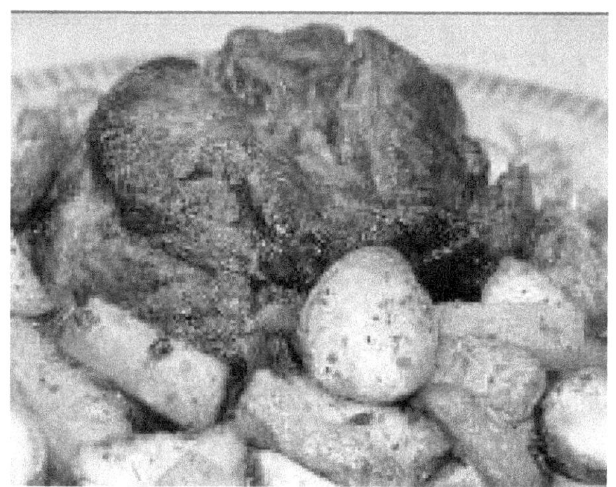

Prep time: 15 mins

Servings: 3

Ingredients:

- 1 ¼ lbs. shoulder or chuck roast

- 2 large carrots

- 2 large potatoes

- ½ large onion

- ½ tsp. black pepper

- 2 sprigs rosemary

- ¼ cup red wine

- ½ tsp. salt

- ½ tsp. pepper

Preparation:

1. In a large oven-roasting bag, place the carrots, potatoes and onion together.

2. Place the chuck or shoulder roast over the layer of vegetables.

3. Combine the wine, pepper, salt and rosemary together in a small mixing bowl.

4. Pour the seasoning over the meat.

5. Seal the bag with the tie and make a tiny slit on the top.

6. Place the sealed oven-roasting bag on a 1-inch rack with the side with the slit facing up.

7. Set the oven on the '7' setting and roast for about 4 to 5 hours.

8. Remove the oven-roasting and place on a tray.

9. Rest meat for about 5 minutes before cutting open the bag.

10.	Slice the roasted meat and serve hot topped with the cooking jus and with the roasted vegetables on the side.

11.	Enjoy!

Nutritional Info:

Calories: 290

Total Fat: 8g

Carbs: 37g

Protein: 18g

Spicy Beef Jerky

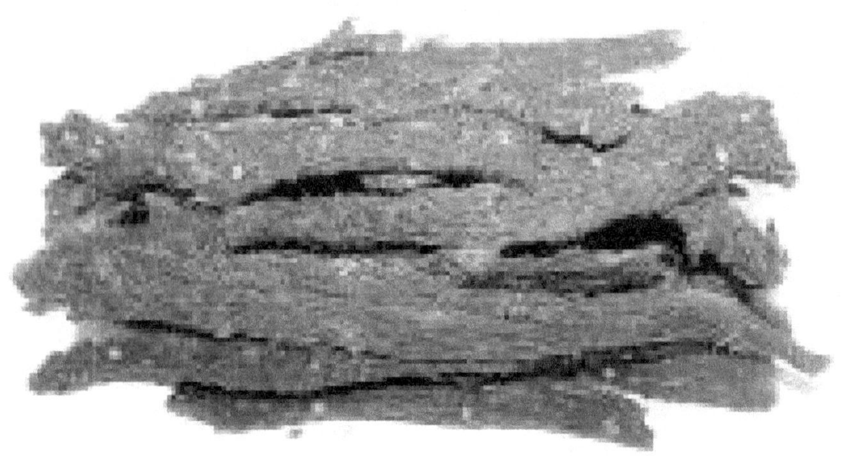

Prep time: 10 mins

Servings: 5

Ingredients:

- 1 lb. beef steak

- 1/8 c. soy sauce

- 1 tbsp. Worcestershire sauce

- 1 tsp. liquid smoke

- 1 tbsp. light brown sugar

- 1 tsp. sea salt

- 1 tsp. ground black pepper

- ½ tsp. powdered garlic

- ½ tsp. powdered onion

- ½ tsp. cayenne pepper

- ½ tsp. paprika

Preparation:

1. Place all ingredients in large recloseable plastic bag or container with a lid. Mix to evenly coat beef strips. Place in refrigerator and marinate overnight (at least 8 hours).

2. Remove beef strips and arrange in liner pan and 3-inch rack.

3. Cook on Power level 4 (175 degrees F) for 3 to 3 ½ hours.

4. Serve Immediately.

5. Enjoy!

Nutritional Info:

Calories: 89

Total Fat: 1g

Carbs: 8g

Protein: 12g

Barbeque Lamb Skewers

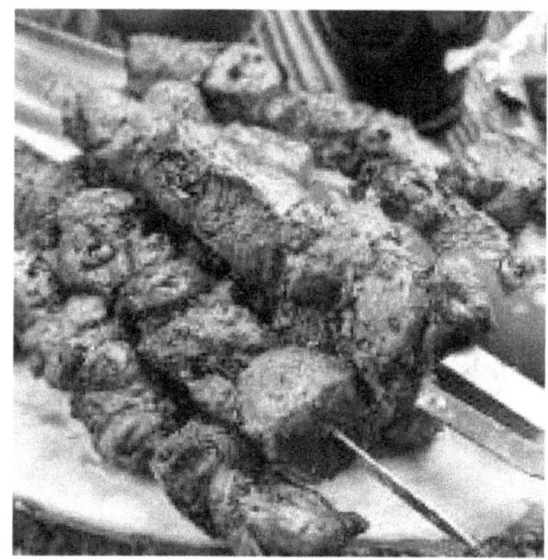

Prep time: 10 minutes

Servings: 2

Ingredients:

- 1lb. lamb leg
- ½ quartered red onion
- ½ large green bell pepper
- 4 large white mushrooms
- Barbeque sauce
- 2 Roma tomatoes

Preparation:

1. Divide the lamb cubes, onion quarters and green pepper pieces into two equal portions.

2. Thread the lamb cubes, onion quarters, green pepper pieces, mushrooms and Roma tomatoes on to bamboo or metal skewers in an alternating pattern of meat and vegetables.

3. Place the prepared skewers on the 3-inch rack and lightly brush the barbeque sauce over them.

4. Grill on the high setting for about 12 to 15 minutes.

5. Flip the skewers over and again brush them with the barbeque sauce.

6. Continue grilling for another 8 to 10 minutes.

7. Serve hot with barbeque sauce on the side.

8. Enjoy!

Nutritional Info:

Calories: 287

Total fat: 12g

Total carbs: 11g

Protein: 33g

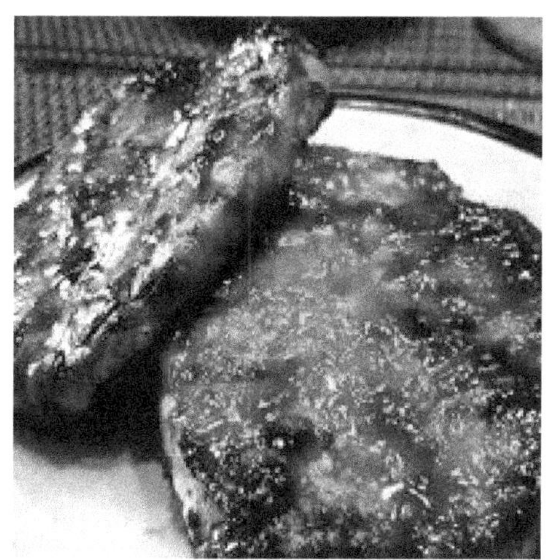

Prep time: 10 mins

Servings: 4

Ingredients:

- 4 pork chops

- ¼ c. cider vinegar

- 3 c. honey

- 2 minced garlic cloves

- ½ tsp. ground ginger

- 1 ½ tbsps. soy sauce

- ½ tsp. ground black pepper

Preparation:

1. In a mixing bowl, add all ingredients apart from pork chops.

2. Pour into large zipper-lock bag and add pork chops. Seal and shake for coating pork chops. Place in refrigerator for a minimum of 1 hour.

3. Place pork chops on 4-inch rack. Cook on High (350 degrees F) for 5 mins each side or till the pork reaches an internal temp of 160 degrees.

4. Serve Hot.

5. Enjoy!

Nutritional Info:

Calories: 204.3

Total Fat: 5.7g

Total carbs: 18.4g

Protein: 19.9g

Hot and Spicy Chorizo Burgers

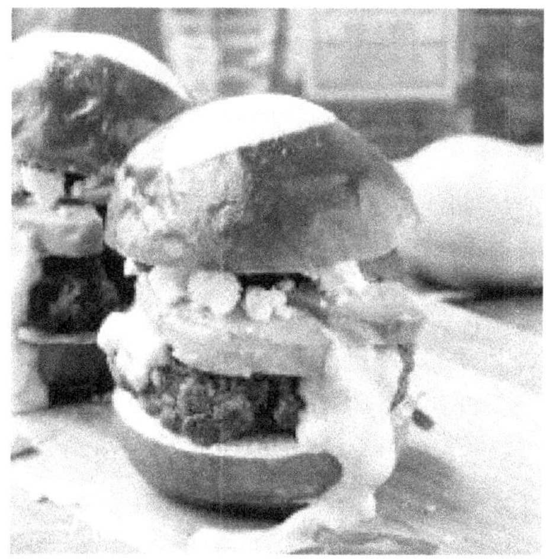

Prep time: 10 mins

Servings: 2

Ingredients:

- ¼ lb. chorizo

- ½ tsp. ground cumin

- ¼ lb. lean ground beef

- ¼ tsp. ground coriander

- 2 chopped garlic cloves

- 1 tbsp. chopped cilantro

- Kosher salt

- ¼ c. mayonnaise

- Black pepper

- ¾ tbsps. hot sauce

- 1 tbsp. olive oil

- ½ tsp. fresh lime juice

- 2 slices pepper jack cheese

- Lettuce leaves

- Sliced tomatoes

- 2 hamburger buns

- 1 ripe Hass avocado

Preparation:

1. Place the chorizo, cumin, ½ tablespoon cilantro, salt, beef, coriander, garlic, and pepper in a medium mixing bowl.

2. Divide the mixture into two then make 2 patties that are about 3-inches wide and about 1-inch thick each.

3. Place the prepared patties on a 3-inch rack and grill on the 'HI' setting for 8 to 10 minutes on each side.

4. While the patties cook in the oven, combine the remaining cilantro with the mayonnaise, lime juice, pepper, hot sauce and salt in a small mixing bowl. Keep aside.

5. Once the patties are done and place a slice of cheese on each patty. Continue baking on the 'HI' setting for another minute or until the cheese melts.

6. Spoon the spicy mayonnaise on the bottom buns and place the lettuce, tomato slices and avocado slices on it.

7. Top with the cheese topped burger patties and cover with the top half of the burger bun.

8. Serve hot.

9. Enjoy!

Nutritional Info:

Calories: 273

Total fat: 23.0g

Carbs: 1.1g

Protein: 14.5g

Apple Butter Pork Tenderloin

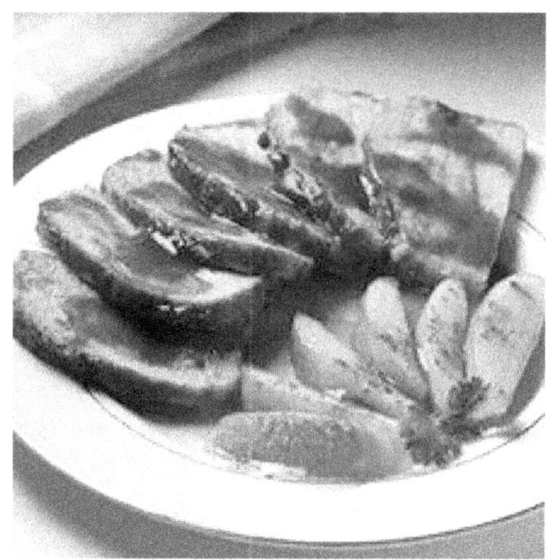

Prep time: 10 mins

Servings: 4

Ingredients:

- ¼ tsp. dried thyme

- 1 lb. pork tenderloin

- 1/8 tsp. mustard powder

- 2 minced garlic cloves

- 4 tbsps. soy sauce

- 4 tbsps. sherry wine

- Ingredients for the sauce:

- 6 tbsps. apple butter

- 1 tbsp. sherry wine

- 1 tbsp. soy sauce

- ¾ tsp. garlic salt

Preparation:

1. Combine thyme, garlic, mustard powder, sherry, and soy sauce in a gallon-size zipper-lock bag. Add tenderloin then marinate in the refrigerator for a minimum of 4 hours, preferably overnight.

2. Remove tenderloin from bag, discard marinade, and place in roasting pan.

3. Combine the apple butter, sherry, soy sauce, and garlic salt in a bowl.

4. Cover pork with the apple butter mixture.

5. Place tenderloin on the 4-inch rack and cook on High (350 °C) for 10 - 12 mins each side.

6. Serve Hot.

7. Enjoy!

Nutritional Info:

Calories: 172

Total carbs: 9g

Total Fat: 4.5g

Protein: 23g

Rib Roast

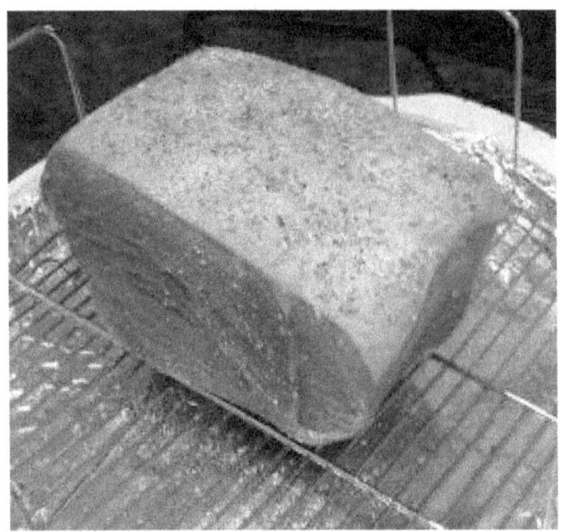

Prep time:

Servings: 4

Ingredients:

- 2 ½ lbs. standing rib roast

- ½ tsp. sea salt

- ½ tsp. powdered onion

- ½ tsp. ground black pepper

Preparation:

1. Combine the sea salt, onion powder and black pepper together in a medium mixing bowl.

2. Put the standing rib roast on the cutting board.

3. Sprinkle the prepared rub over the rib roast and rub it in using your fingers. Make sure you rub the spice rub in especially around the boney areas.

4. Place the spice rub coated rib roast on a 1-inch rack with its rib side down.

5. Grill on the 'HI' setting for about 14 to 16 minutes per pound of ribs, for rare done ribs.

6. Remove the ribs oven and rest them for about 10 mins before slicing.

7. Serve hot with hot sauce or barbeque sauce on the side.

8. Enjoy!

Nutritional Info:

Calories: 354.0

Total Fat: 25.9g

Total carbs 0.0 g

Protein: 28.0

Sweet and Spicy Baby Back Ribs

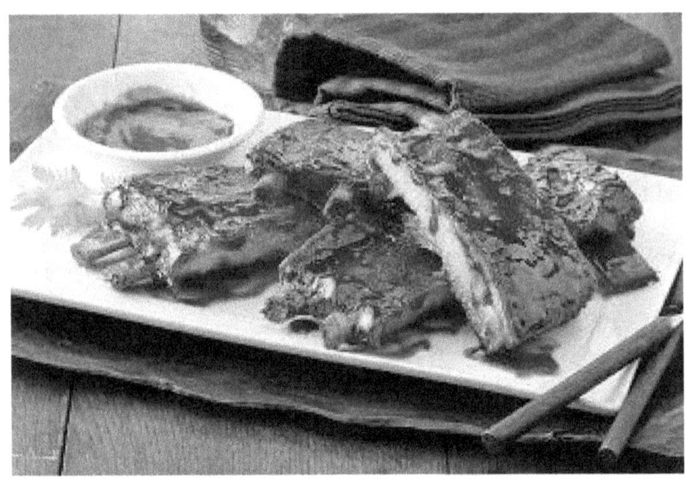

Prep time: 10 mins

Servings: 6

Ingredients:

- ½ c. paprika
- ¼ c. granulated onion
- ½ c. granulated garlic
- ¼ c. kosher salt
- ¼ c. cumin
- ¼ c. black pepper
- 2 tbsps. chipotle or ancho pepper

- ¼ c.

- 2 c. brown sugar

- 6 c. water

- 2 slabs baby back ribs

- 4 tbsps. liquid smoke

Preparation:

1. Combine the paprika, granulated onion, kosher salt, ground cumin, ground black pepper, chipotle or ancho pepper, granulated garlic cayenne pepper and mustard powder in a medium-sized mixing bowl. Whisk well till all ingredients are well mixed.

2. Add brown sugar to the spice mix then mix well to combine.

3. Spoon the prepared spice rub on the slab of baby ribs and coat the baby ribs on all sides. Make sure that you rub the spice rub into all the boney and fatty areas of the baby ribs.

4. Combine the liquid smoke and water together in a mixing bowl. Whisk well until well combined and pour it into the lined pan.

5. Place spice-rubbed baby rib slabs on the 1-inch rack.

6. Set your NuWave oven to the '5' setting and grill your baby ribs for about 90 minutes.

7. Carefully open the dome of the oven, taking care so that you do not burn yourself, and turn the ribs over using metal tongs.

8. Continue grilling the baby ribs for another 3 to 3 and half hours.

9. Once the ribs are done, remove the ribs from oven and rest for 10 mins.

10. Serve hot.

11. Enjoy!

Nutritional Info:

Calories: 304

Total Fat: 18g

Total Carbs: 0g

Protein: 18g

Seafood and Poultry Recipes

Citrus Baked Salmon

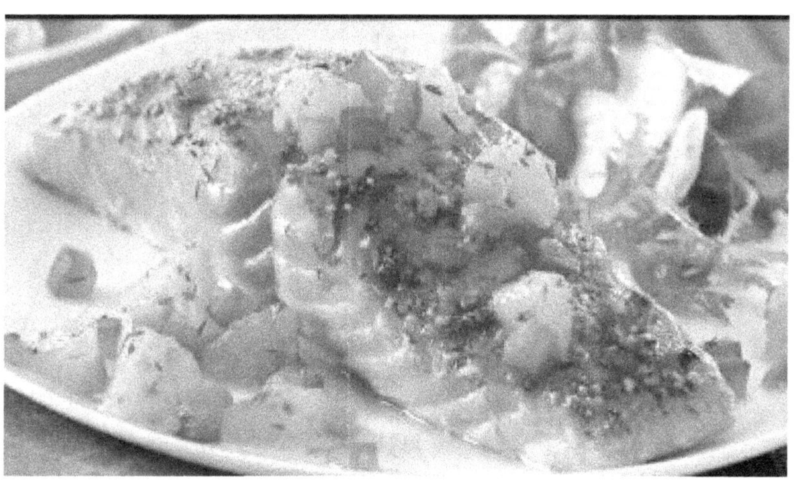

Prep time: 5 mins

Servings: 4

Ingredients:

- 4 slices lemon
- 4 slices orange
- 4 salmon fillets
- Salt
- Black pepper
- 2 tbsps. chopped dill

- 2 tbsps. tomatoes

- 1 tbsp. virgin olive oil

- 2/3 c. rice wine vinegar

Preparation:

1. Place lemon and orange slices, side by side, in the bottom of a shallow baking dish that will fit in NuWave oven (10 x10). Place each salmon fillet across the citrus slices. Sprinkle with pepper and salt.

2. In a bowl, combine dill, sun-dried tomatoes, olive oil, and rice wine vinegar. Drizzle mixture over salmon fillets.

3. Place on 1-inch rack and cook on High power (350 °C) for 7-8 mins or till salmon is cooked through.

4. Serve Immediately.

5. Enjoy!

Nutritional Info:

Calories: 272.0

Total Fat: 12.6g

Total carbs: 5.4g

Protein: 32.5g

Tuna Noodle Casserole

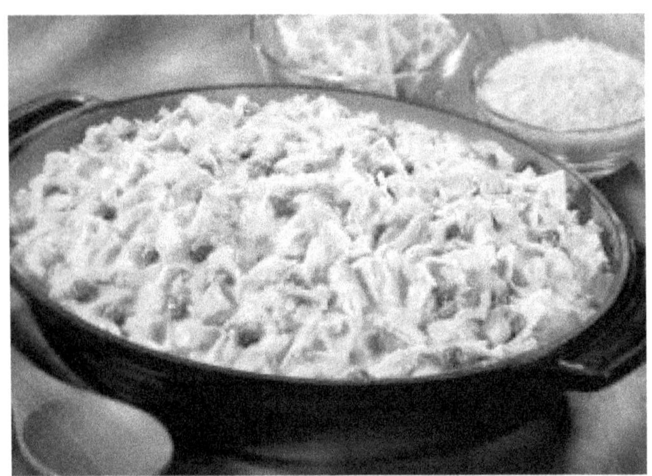

Prep time: 5 mins

Servings: 6

Ingredients:

- 5 oz. can tuna

- 10½ oz. creamy mushroom soup

- 1 c. egg noodles

- ¼ c. cold water

- ½ c. frozen peas or green beans

- 2 tbsps. Breadcrumbs

- ¼ c. sour cream

- ½ c. shredded Cheddar cheese

Preparation:

1. Place the tuna, sour cream, green beans or peas, about 6 tablespoons cheese, cream of mushroom soup, and cooked noodles together in a medium mixing bowl.

2. Mix well until it forms a cohesive mixture.

3. Pour the prepared mix into an 8-inch ovenproof dish.

4. Place the ovenproof dish on the 1-inch rack and cook on the 'HI' setting for about 18 to 22 minutes.

5. Once the timer is up, add the remaining cheese and breadcrumbs on the top of the semi-set casserole.

6. Bake on the 'HI' setting for another 2 to 3 minutes or until the cheese melts and gets light brown.

7. Once done, remove the casserole oven and allow cooling for about 7 - 10 mins before serving.

8. Enjoy!

Nutritional Info:

Calories: 267

Total Fat: 11g

Carbs: 25g

Protein: 19g

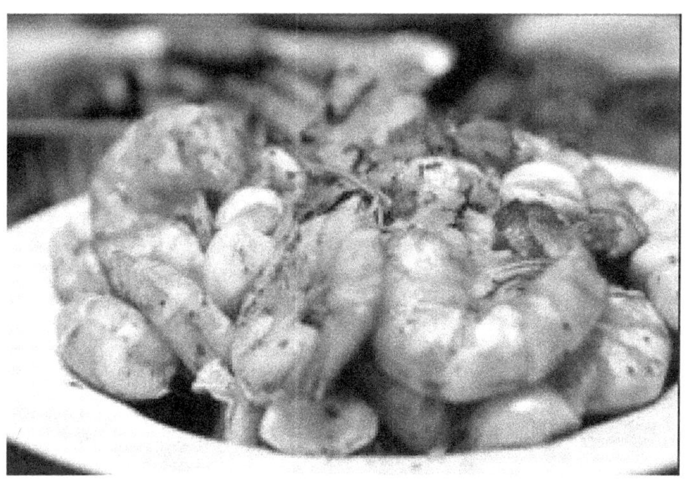

Prep time: 15 mins

Servings: 4

Ingredients:

- 3 tbsps. lime juice

- ¼ c. virgin olive oil

- 2 garlic cloves

- 2 tbsps. tequila

- ½ tsp. ground cumin

- ½ tsp. cayenne pepper

- Salt

- Black

- 1 lb. extra-large shrimp

Preparation:

1. In a mixing bowl, whisk together lime juice, virgin olive oil, garlic, cumin, cayenne pepper, salt, tequila and pepper. Add shrimp and marinate for 2-3 hours in the refrigerator.

2. Line bottom of NuWave Oven with foil.

3. Place shrimp on the 4-inch rack. Cook on High Power (350 degrees F) for 3 mins. Flip shrimp over and cook for another 3 mins or until shrimp are opaque.

4. Serve Immediately.

5. Enjoy!

6. **Nutritional Info:**

Calories: 270

Total Fat: 13g

Total Carbs: 6g

Protein: 19 g

Crab Cakes

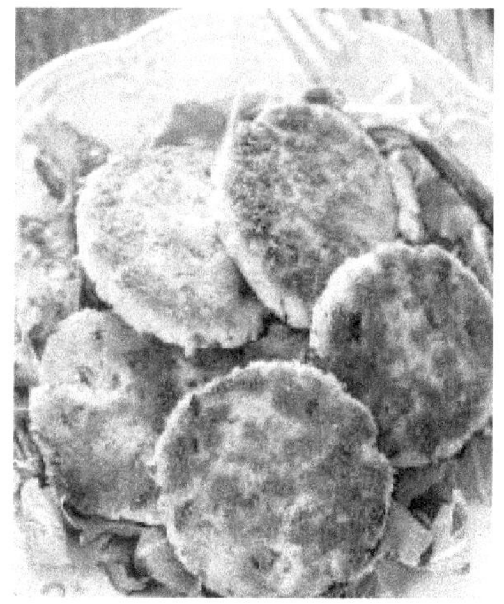

Prep time: 5 mins

Servings: 4

Ingredients:

- 2/3 c. panko breadcrumbs
- 1 tbsp. chopped parsley
- 2 tbsps. chopped green onions
- ½ tsp. Old Bay seasoning
- ½ tsp. Worcestershire sauce
- ¼ tsp. sea salt
- ¼ tsp. cayenne pepper

- 1tsp. lemon juice

- 2 ½ tbsps. mayonnaise

- 1 large egg

- 8 oz. lump crabmeat

- 1 lemon

- 1 tsp. Dijon mustard

Preparation:

1. In a large bowl, combine 1/3 cup breadcrumbs, parsley, green onions, Old Bay seasoning, Worcestershire sauce, salt, cayenne pepper, lemon juice, mayonnaise, mustard, and egg. Add crabmeat and stir until just combined.

2. Place remaining breadcrumbs in shallow dish. Form crab mixture into 4 equal size patties. Coat each side with breadcrumbs.

3. Place foil on 3-inch rack. Spray lightly with cooking spray. Place patties on foil. Bake on High Power (350 °C) for 6 mins. Lip and cook extra 6 minutes.

4. Serve immediately.

5. Enjoy!

Nutritional Info:

Calories: 260

Total Fat: 18g

Carbs: 13g

Protein: 11g

Roasted Shrimp with a Herbed Salsa

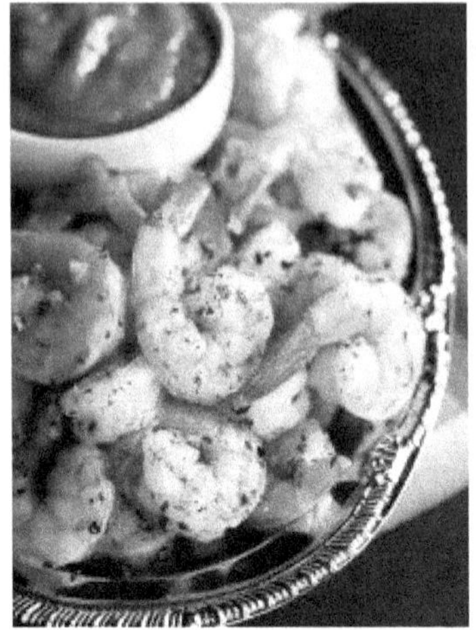

Prep time: 5 mins

Servings: 2

Ingredients:

- ¾ lb. large shrimp

- 3 sliced garlic cloves

- 1 red Serrano pepper

- 1 bay leaf

- ½ lemon

- ¼ c. olive oil

- Ingredients for the Herb Salsa:

- 2 tbsps. chopped cilantro

- ½ tbsp. grated lemon zest

- 2 tbsps. chopped flat-leaf parsley

- ½ tbsp. virgin olive oil

- Pepper

- Kosher salt

Preparation:

1. Place the shrimp and Serrano pepper halves in an ovenproof dish, along with the bay leaf, garlic and virgin olive oil.

2. Mix lightly till all the ingredients are well coated with virgin olive oil.

3. Place the baking dish on the 3-inch rack.

4. Cook on the 'HI' setting for about 3 to 5 minutes.

5. While the shrimp cooks, prepare the salsa.

6. Combine the cilantro, lemon zest and parsley together in a small mixing bowl.

7. Add salt nd pepper to taste.

8. Pour the olive oil over the salsa and let it stand for a few minutes before mixing it up.

9. When the shrimp is done, pour in the lemon juice and mix well to coat.

10.   Serve the shrimp hot, topped with the prepared salsa.

11.   Enjoy!

Nutritional Info:

Calories: 100

Fat: 0g

Carbs: 0g

Protein: 18g

Chicken Parmesan

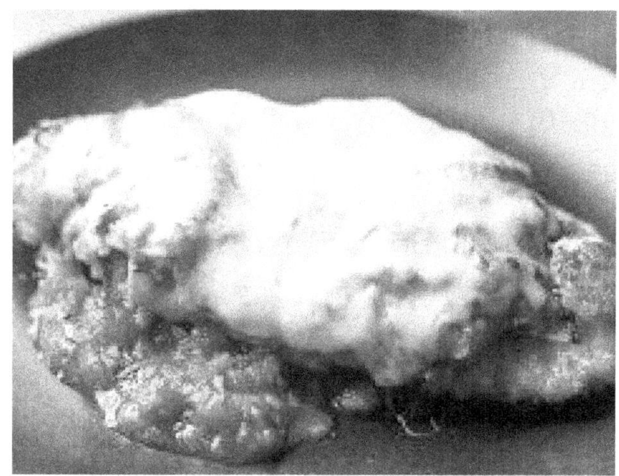

Prep time: 10 mins

Servings: 2

Ingredients:

- 10 oz. chicken breasts

- ½ c. seasoned panko breadcrumbs

- 2 eggs

- ½ c. flour

- ¼ tbsp. Pepper

- ½ tbsp. kosher salt

- 14oz. marinara sauce

- 2 slices provolone cheese

Preparation:

1. Crack open the eggs on a shallow bowl then season lightly with salt and pepper. Whisk well.

2. Put flour in another shallow plate and season it to taste.

3. Finally, place the seasoned panko breadcrumbs in another shallow flat plate.

4. Make light indentions on the chicken breasts with a sharp knife, making sure that you don't cut through.

5. Dip the chicken breasts into the seasoned flour.

6. Then dip the flour coated chicken into the eggs.

7. Finally dip the flour and egg coated chicken into the plate with the breadcrumbs and lightly press until the breadcrumbs stick to the chicken breasts.

8. Place the breadcrumb encrusted chicken on a 3-inch rack and back on the 'HI' setting for about 15 to 17 minutes per side.

9. Place a slice of provolone on each chicken breast and continue baking on the 'HI' setting for another 2 to 3 minutes, or until the cheese melts.

10.   Put the chicken breasts on serving plates then slather the marinara sauce over them.

11.   Serve hot.

12.   Enjoy!

Nutritional Info:

Calories: 254

Total Fat: 12.38g

Total carbs: 12.18g

Protein: 22.83g

Oven Fried Chicken Wings

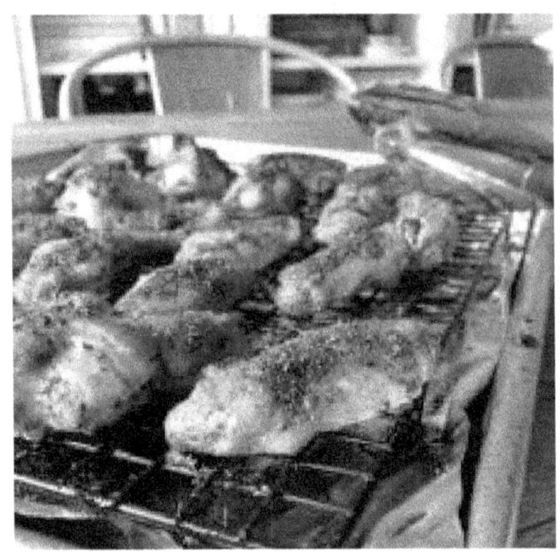

Prep time: 5 mins

Servings: 4

Ingredients:

- Cooking spray

- 1/3 c. grated Parmesan cheese

- 1/3 c. panko-style breadcrumbs

- 1/8 tsp. powdered garlic

- 1/8 tsp. powdered onion

- 1/3 c. breadcrumbs

- 1/8 tsp. ground black pepper

- ¼ c. melted butter

- 1 ½ lbs. chicken wings

- Salt

Preparation:

1. In a baking sheet, spray with cooking spray.

2. Mix Parmesan cheese, garlic powder, onion powder, black pepper, breadcrumbs and salt.

3. Dip chicken wings one at a time into melted butter and then into bread mixture until thoroughly covered. Arrange wings in single layer on the baking sheet.

4. Place on 1-inch rack and cook on High power (350 degrees F) for 10 mins. Flip wings over and cook for another 10-12 mins until no longer pink in centre and juices run clear. Remove promptly from NuWave Oven.

5. Serve Hot.

6. Enjoy!

Nutritional Info:

Calories: 370.8

Total Fat: 22.6g

Total carbs: 11.8g

Protein: 27.8g

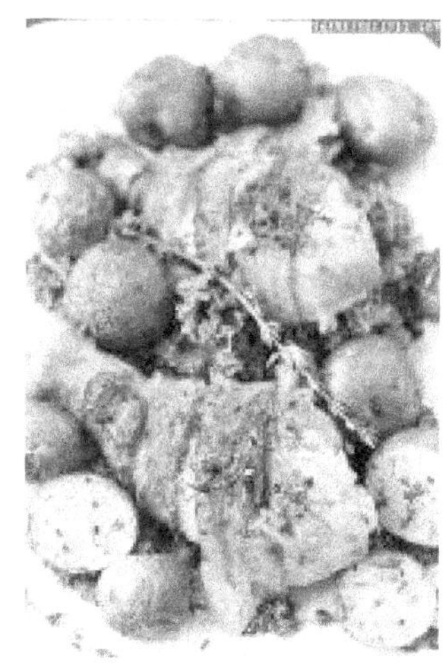

Prep time: 10 mins

Servings: 4

Ingredients:

- 4 chicken thighs

- 8 slices bacon

- 1 lb. baby red potatoes

- 4 bone-in chicken drumsticks

- 1 tbsp. dried basil

- ½ tbsp. garlic powder

- ½ tbsp. adobo seasoning

- ½ tbsp. black pepper

- 1 tsp. salt

Preparation:

1. Wrap each piece of chicken with one slice of bacon.

2. Line bottom of NuWave Oven with foil.

3. Arrange chicken in centre of 4-inch rack. Place potatoes around chicken on rack.

4. In a mixing bowl, mix garlic powder, black pepper, adobo seasoning, basil, and salt. Sprinkle seasoning mixture over chicken and potatoes.

5. Cook on High Power (350 degrees F) for 10 minutes. Turn chicken and potatoes and cook for another10 minutes or until chicken is fully cooked and potatoes are tender.

6. Serve Hot.

7. Enjoy!

Nutritional Info:

Calories: 601.0

Total Fat: 14.8g

Total carbs: 74.8g

Protein: 41.9g

Garlic Ginger Chicken Wings

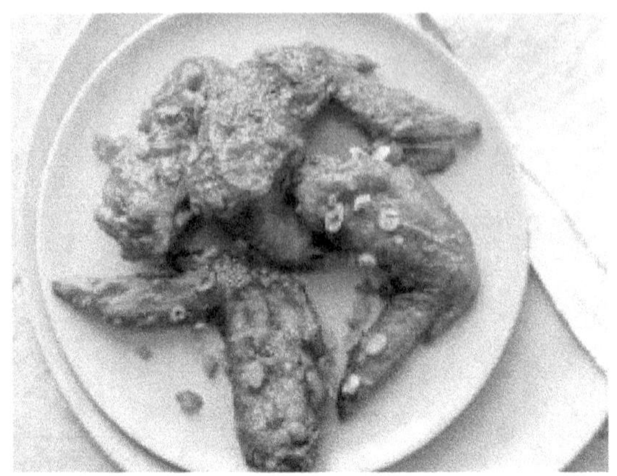

Prep time: 10 mins

Servings: 4

Ingredients:

- 1½ tbsps. vegetable oil

- Salt

- Black pepper

- 1 tbsp. Frank's Red Hot Sauce

- 1 ½ lbs. chicken wings

- 1/3 c. flour

- For glaze:

- 3 crushed garlic

- 1 tbsp. Asian chilli pepper sauce

- ¼ c. rice wine vinegar

- 1 tbsp. minced ginger

- ¼ c. light brown sugar

- 1½ tbsps. soy sauce

Preparation:

1. In a large mixing bowl, combine Frank's Red Hot Sauce, vegetable oil, salt and pepper. Add chicken wings and toss to coat thoroughly.

2. Place coated wings in large zip lock bag. Add flour, seal bag and shake until wings are coated with flour.

3. Place wings on the 4-inch rack and cook on High power (350 degrees F) for 10 minutes. Turn wings over and cook for an additional 8 minutes.

4. In a large bowl, whisk together all ingredients for glaze. Place wings in glaze and toss to coat evenly. Place wings back on the 4-inch rack and cook on High power for an additional 5 mins.

5. Remove from oven then serve.

6. Enjoy!

Nutritional Info:

Calories: 230

Fat: 7.5g

Carbohydrates: 21.1g

Protein: 18.8g

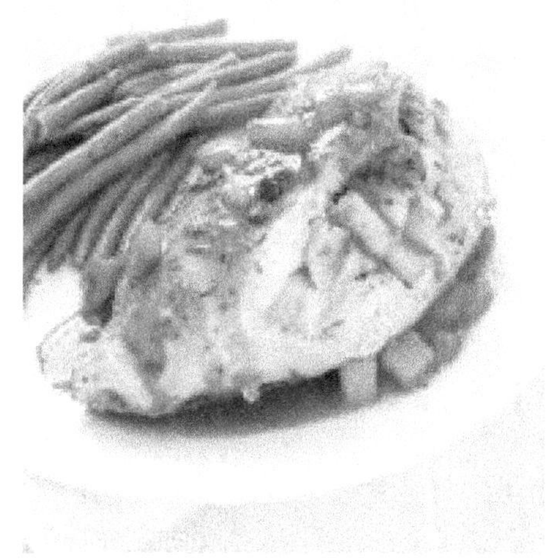

Prep time: 10 mins

Servings: 4

Ingredients:

- 2 chicken breasts

- 1 large apple

- 2 tbsps. Cheddar cheese, shredded

- 1½ tbsps. Panko-style breadcrumbs

- 2 tbsps. Chopped pecans,

- 2 tbsps. Light brown sugar

- 1 tsp. cinnamon

- 1 tsp. curry powder

Preparation:

1. In a bowl, add apple, cheese, breadcrumbs, pecans, brown sugar, cinnamon, and curry powder.

2. Pound chicken breasts between waxed paper sheets till thick.

3. Spread half the apple mixture on every chicken breast. Roll the chicken up and secure with toothpicks.

4. Place chicken on the 4-inch rack and cook on High power for 12 mins. Flip over and cook for another 10-12 mins.

5. Serve Hot.

6. Enjoy!

Nutritional Info:

Calories: 1016

Carbs: 18g

Fat: 44g

Protein: 121g

Vegetable Recipes

Sweet Potato Casserole

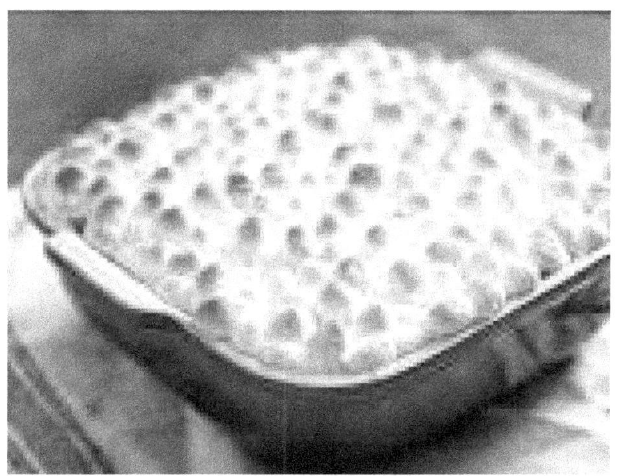

Prep time: 15 mins

Servings: 6

Ingredients:

- 2 c. sweet potatoes

- ¼ c. melted butter

- 1½ tbsps. milk

- ¼ c. honey

- vanilla

- 1 large egg

- ¼ c. sugar

- ¼ c. wheat flour

- 2 tbsps. butter

- ½ c. chopped pecans

Preparation:

1. Spray baking sheet with cooking spray.

2. In a mixing bowl, add milk, honey, sweet potatoes, vanilla, melted butter, and egg.

3. In a mixing bowl, mix brown sugar and flour. Cut in 3 tablespoons butter till crumbly. Add pecans and mix.

4. Sprinkle the mixture over sweet potatoes.

5. Place on 1-inch rack and cook for 25-30 mins at 350°C (High) or until golden brown.

6. Serve Immediately.

Nutritional Info:

Calories: 310

Total Fat: 13g

Carbs: 49g

Protein: 3g

Roasted Garlic Mushrooms

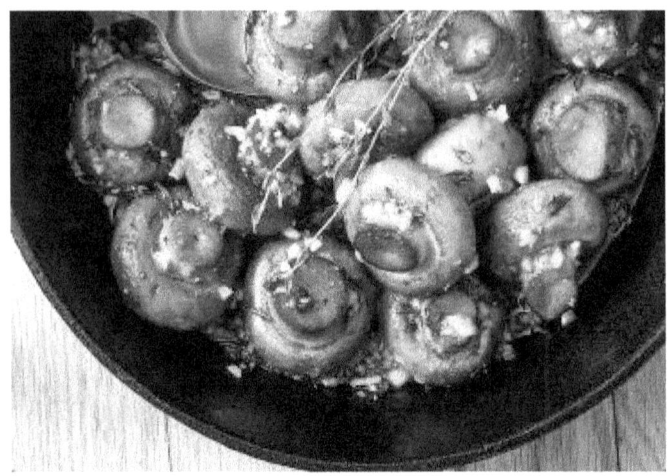

Prep time: 5 mins

Servings: 2

Ingredients:

- 8oz. package crimini or button mushrooms
- 2 chopped garlic cloves
- 2 tbsps. olive oil
- 1 tbsp. chopped thyme
- Black pepper
- Salt

Preparation:

1. Place the olive oil, garlic and fresh thyme together in a small bowl. Whisk till well combined.

2. Add pepper and salt to taste.

3. Pour the marinade on the mushrooms and mix well until the mushrooms are properly coated.

4. Place marinated mushrooms directly onto the lined pan.

5. Roast on the 'HI' setting for about 20 to 25 minutes.

6. Serve hot. Enjoy!

Nutritional Info:

Calories: 360

Total Fat: 18g

Carbs: 44g

Protein: 6g

Roasted Cauliflower, Olives and Chickpeas

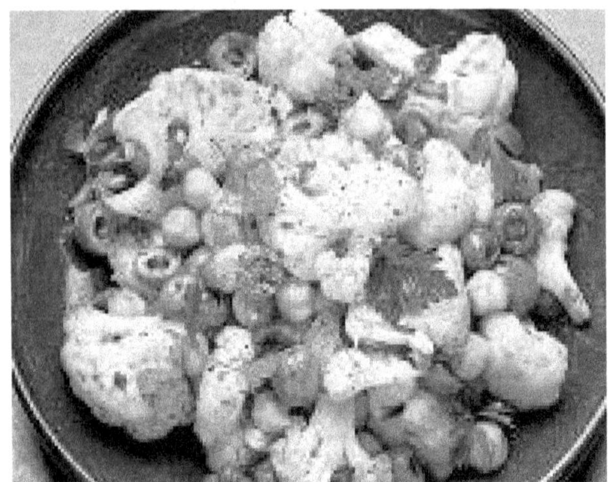

Prep time: 5 mins

Servings: 3

Ingredients:

- 3 c. cauliflower florets

- 4 chopped garlic cloves

- ½ c. Spanish green olives

- 15 oz. chickpeas, rinsed and drained

- ¼ tsp crushed red pepper

- 1 ½ tbsps. olive oil

- 1 ½ tbsps. parsley

- ¼ tsp. salt

Preparation:

1. Place the cauliflower florets, garlic, Spanish green olives, chickpeas, crushed red pepper, parsley and salt in a large bowl.

2. Pour oil over the ingredients, then let it stand for about 2 to 3 minutes.

3. Toss until all the ingredients are well coated in the olive oil.

4. Place the olive oil coated ingredients at the bottom of a lined pan in a single even layer.

5. Cook on 'HI' setting for about 22 to 24 minutes.

6. Serve hot with your preferred condiment on the side.

Nutritional Info:

Calories: 176

Fat: 10.1g

Protein: 4.2g

Carbs: 17.6g

Fruit and Vegetable Skewers

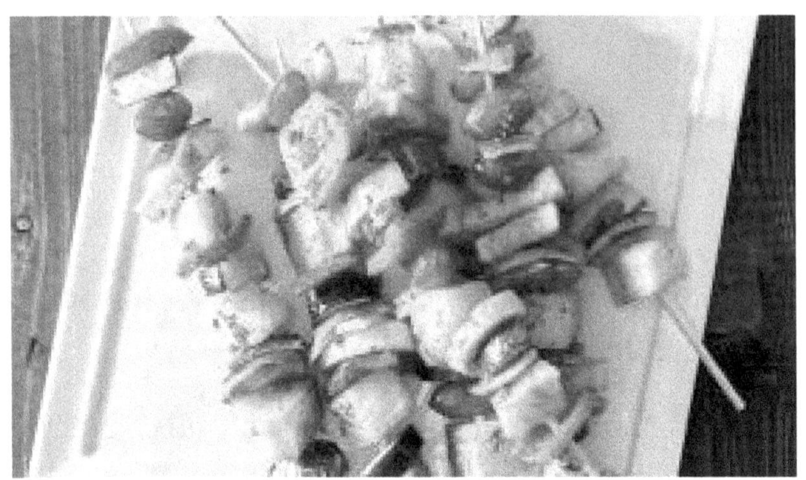

Prep time: 5 mins

Servings: 4

Ingredients:

- ¼ c. virgin olive oil

- 3 tbsps. lemon juice

- 1 minced garlic clove

- 2 tbsps. chopped parsley

- ½ tsp. salt

- ½ tsp. black pepper

- 1 sliced zucchini

- 1 sliced yellow squash

- ½ red bell pepper

- ½ c. cherry tomatoes

- ½ c. pineapple chunks

- 4 wooden skewers

Preparation:

1. Mix virgin olive oil, garlic, parsley, lemon juice, pepper, and salt in a bowl. Pour into large resealable plastic bag. Add zucchini, squash, bell pepper, and tomatoes. Seal bag, shake to coat vegetables, and place in refrigerator for a minimum of 1 hour.

2. Remove vegetables from marinade and thread onto skewers, along with pineapple, alternating among each item.

3. Line bottom of NuWave Oven with foil for easier clean-up.

4. Place skewers on the 4-inch rack. Cook on High Power (350°C) for 8 mins.

5. Flip skewers over and cook for another 6-8 mins until veggies are desired level of doneness.

6. Remove from NuWave Oven, transfer to a plate, and serve.

7. Enjoy!

Nutritional Info:

Calories: 173.4

Total Fat: 2.8 g

Total carbs: 36.5g

Protein: 5.0g

Roasted sweet potatoes with rosemary

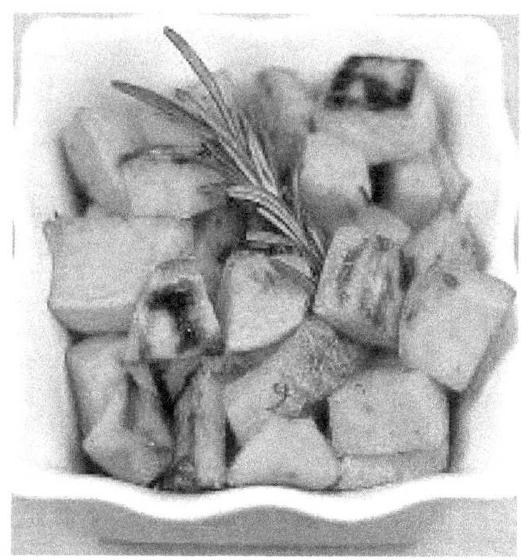

Prep time: 10 mins

Servings: 4

Ingredients:

- 1 ½ lbs. cubed sweet potatoes

- 1 tsp. olive oil

- 1 dash chopped rosemary

- 1 dash lemon juice

Preparation:

1. In a bowl, toss sweet potatoes with oil. Evenly spread on the 10-inch baking sheet, sprinkle with rosemary. Place on 1-inch rack and back on High

power (350 degrees F) for 12 minutes. Flip sweet
potatoes over and cook an additional 10 minutes.

2. Drizzle with lemon juice and serve.

Nutritional Info:

Calories: 114

Total fat: 0g

Carbs: 27g

Protein: 2g

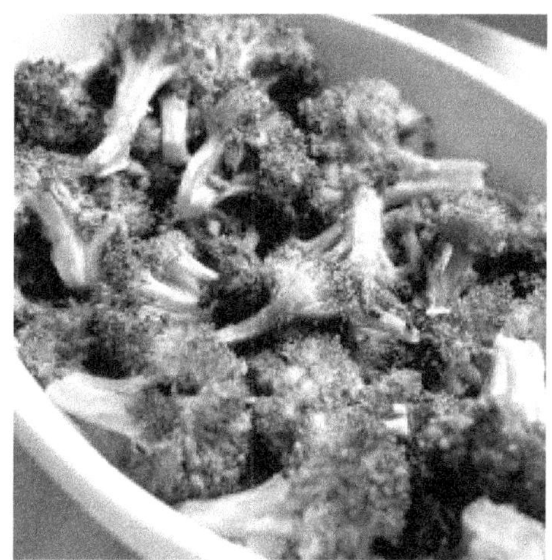

Prep time: 10 mins

Servings: 4

Ingredients:

- 3 garlic cloves, minced

- 2 tsps. Virgin olive oil

- 1 tsp. sea salt

- ½ tsp. black pepper

- 1 broccoli head

- ½ tsp. lemon juice

Preparation:

1. In a mixing bowl, add oil, salt, garlic and black pepper. Add broccoli. Mix to coat. Evenly scatter broccoli on the 10-inch baking sheet.

2. Place on1-inch rack and roast on High power (350 degrees F) for about 10 mins. Flip florets and cook another 5-7 mins or until fork tender.

3. Plate and drizzle lemon juice. Serve at once.

Nutritional Info:

Calories: 141

Carbs: 10g

Fat: 10 g

Protein: 5g

Roasted carrots with garlic

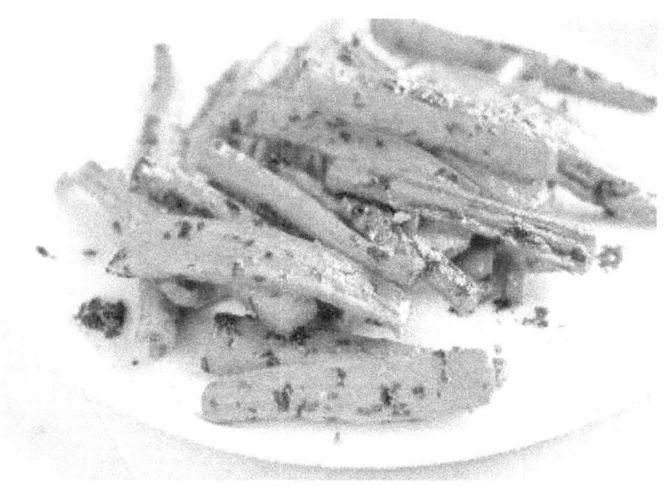

Prep time: 10 mins

Servings: 4

Ingredients:

- 3 tbsps. olive oil
- 2 minced garlic cloves
- Sea salt
- 1 lb. baby carrots

Preparation:

1. In a medium bowl, mix carrots with olive oil, salt and garlic. Spread carrots in single layer on parchment or foil-lined baking sheet.

2. Place on 1-inch rack and cook on High power (350 F) for 15-20 mins until carrots are tender.

Nutritional Info:

Calories: 95.3

Total Fat: 6.9g

Total carbs: 7.6g

Protein: 0.8g

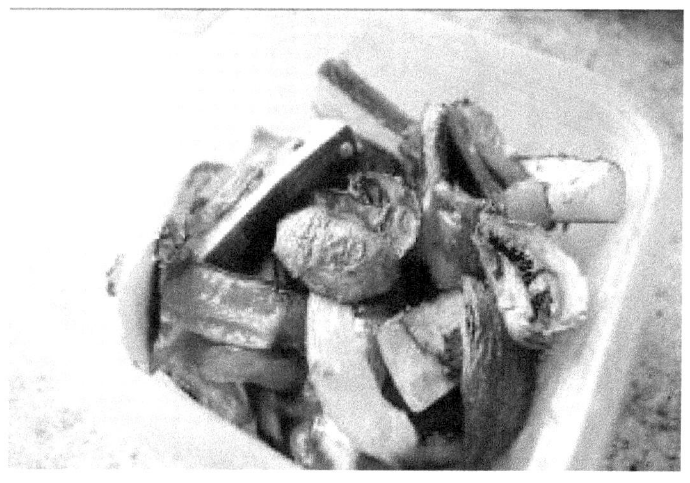

Prep time: 10 mins

Servings: 4

Ingredients:

- 1½ c. cubed butternut squash

- 1 c. chopped broccoli florets

- ½ chopped red onion

- 1 chopped zucchini

- 1 minced garlic clove

- 2 tbsps. virgin olive oil

- 1½ tsps. rosemary

- ½ tsp. sea salt

- 1 tbsp. balsamic vinegar

Preparation:

1. In a mixing bowl, add oil, rosemary, vinegar, pepper, and salt; mix to blend. Mix in the vegetables, mix to coat evenly.

2. Evenly spread on a parchment-lined baking sheet.

3. Place on 1-inch rack and cook on High power (350 degrees F) for about 15 mins. Flip vegetables and cook for another 15 mins or until squash is just softened.

Nutritional Info:

Calories: 148

Total Fat: 4.6g

Total carbs: 25.64g

Protein: 6.61g

Baked macaroni and cheese

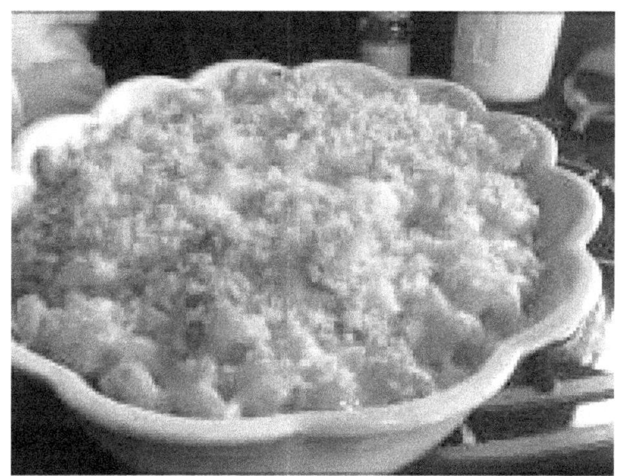

Prep time: 5 mins

Servings: 8

Ingredients:

- 1 lb. cheddar cheese, shredded

- 4 tbsps. butter

- 2 eggs

- 1 tsp. Dijon mustard

- 12 oz. evaporated milk

- 1 lb. elbow macaroni

- Salt

- ½ c. breadcrumbs

- Black pepper

Preparation:

1. Cook macaroni according to package directions.

2. Spray casserole dish with cooking spray.

3. Add all ingredients except for bread crumbs to a casserole dish and mix well to combine. Sprinkle with breadcrumbs.

4. Cover with foil and place pan on 1-inch rack. Bake on High (350 degrees F) for 15-20 minutes. Remove the foil then cook for another 5-10 mins or until golden brown.

Nutritional Info:

Calories: 580

Total Fat: 19g

Carbs: 70g

Protein: 34g

Curried zucchini chips

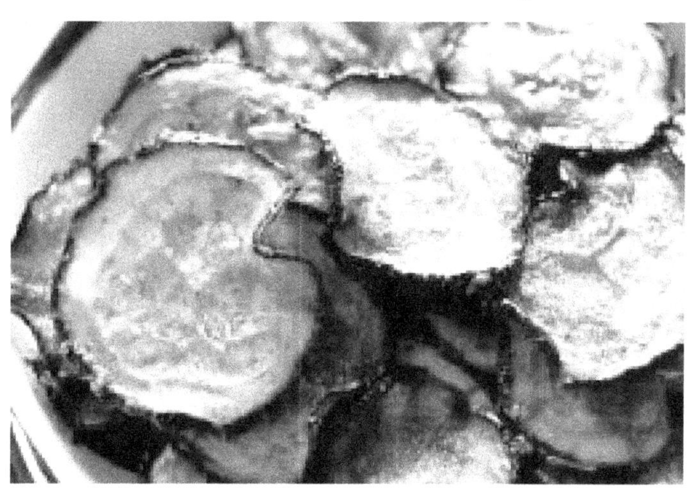

Prep time: 5 mins

Servings: 2

Ingredients:

- 1 medium sliced zucchini

- 1 tbsp. virgin olive oil

- ⅛ tsp. garlic powder

- ¼ tsp. curry powder

- ⅛ tsp. salt

Preparation:

1. Lightly grease paper-lined baking sheet.

2. Arrange zucchini slices in one layer on the baking
    sheet. Sprinkle olive oil and dust with curry
    powder, salt, and garlic powder.

3. Place baking sheet on 1-inch rack and bake on
    High power (350 degrees F) for 12 minutes. Flip
    zucchini over and cook for another 10 mins or till
    very crisp. Cool and store in airtight container

Nutritional Info:

Calories: 15.2

Total carbs: 3.6g

Total Fat: 0.1g

Protein: 0.6g

Dessert Recipes

Lemon-zucchini muffins

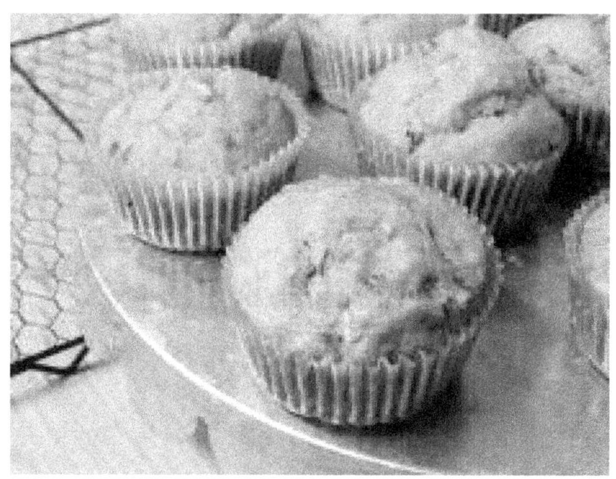

Prep time: 10 mins

Servings: 12

Ingredients:

- 2 c. wheat flour

- ½ c. brown sugar

- 1 tbsp. baking powder

- ¼ tsp. sea salt

- 2 tbsps. olive oil

- ¼ tsp. ground cinnamon

- ¼ tsp. nutmeg

- 1 c. shredded zucchini

- ¾ c. nonfat milk

- 2 tbsps. fresh lemon juice

- Nonstick cooking spray

- 1 egg

Preparation:

1. Prepare 6-muffin tin by spraying with cooking spray or lining with muffin liners.

2. In a mixing bowl, add flour, baking powder, sugar salt, nutmeg and cinnamon

3. In another bowl, mix, milk, zucchini lemon juice, eggs and oil. Mix well.

4. Add zucchini mixture to flour mixture. Stir till just combined. Do not over stir.

5. Pour muffin cups. Place pan on a 1-inch rack and bake for 20 mins at 350 degrees (High) or until light golden brown.

Nutritional Info:

Calories: 370.7

Total Fat: 17.5g

Total carbs: 47.6g

Protein: 7.6 g

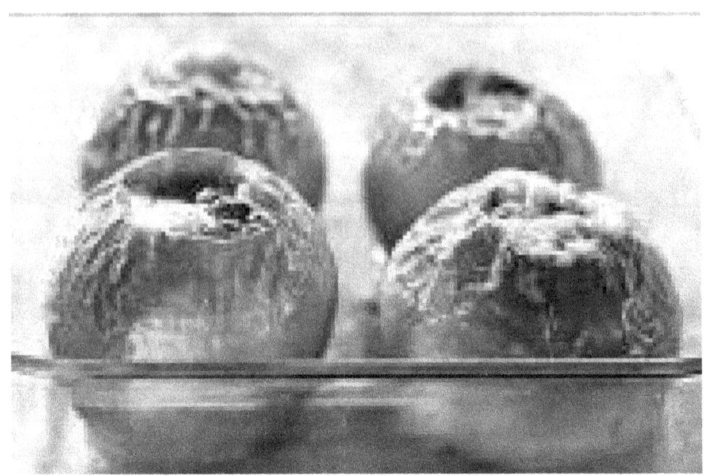

Prep time: 10 mins

Servings: 4

Ingredients:

- 4 large apple

- ¼ c. coconut flakes

- ¼ c. dried cranberries or apricots

- 2 tsps. Grated orange zest

- ½ c. orange juice

- 2 tbsps. brown sugar

Preparations:

1. Cut top off apple and hollow out centre with knife or apple corer. Arrange in non-stick baking pan.

2. In a bowl, combine coconut, cranberries, and orange zest. Divide evenly and fill centres of apples.

3. In a bowl, mix orange juice and brown sugar. Pour over apples.

4. Place pan on a 1-inch rack and cook 5-6 minutes until apples are tender.

5. Serve warm.

Nutritional Info:

Calories: 155.9

Total Fat: 6.7g

Total carbs: 26.1g

Protein: 1.1g

Vitamin A

Carrot cake cookies

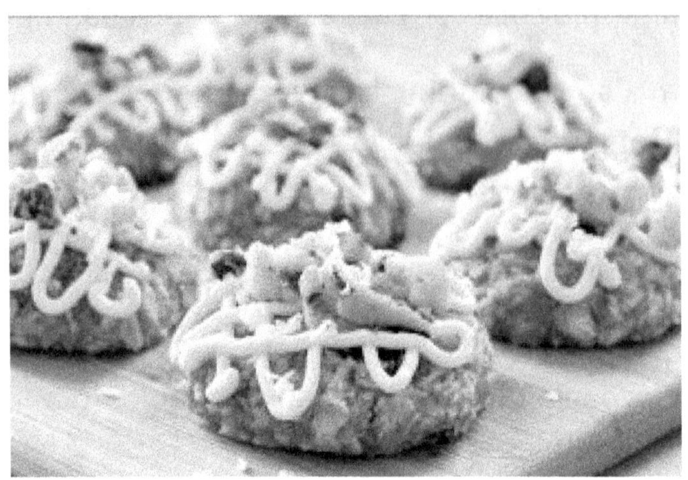

Prep time: 10 mins

Servings: 24

Ingredients:

- ¼ c. brown sugar

- ¼ c. sugar

- ¼ c. oil

- ½ tsp. baking soda

- ¼ c. applesauce or fruit puree

- ¼ tsp. nutmeg

- 1 eggs

- ½ tsp. vanilla

- ½ c. flour

- ½ c. wheat flour

- ½ tsp. baking powder

- 1/8 tsp. sea salt

- ½ tsp. ground cinnamon

- ¼ tsp. ground ginger

- 1 c. old-fashioned rolled oats

- ¾ c. grated carrots

- ½ c. raisins or golden raisins

Preparation:

1. Mix together sugars, oil, applesauce, egg, and vanilla.

2. In another bowl, mix all dry ingredients.

3. Add dry ingredients to wet ingredients. Mix till blended. Toss in carrots and raisins.

4. Drop by teaspoonful onto silicone baking ring or parchment-lined cookie sheet.

5. Place on 1-inch rack and cook at 300 degrees F
   (Level 8) for 12-14 minutes or until golden
   brown.

Nutritional Info:

Calories: 152

Carbs: 20g

Total Fat: 7g

Protein: 1g

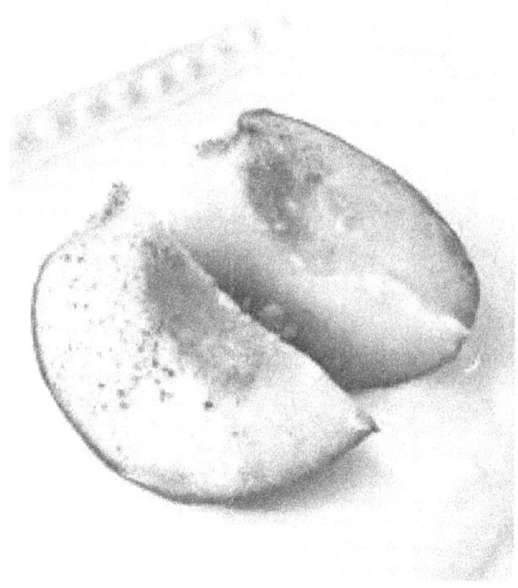

Prep time: 6 mins

Servings: 4

Ingredients:

- 2 peaches

- 1 tbsp. extra-virgin olive oil

- 1 tbsp. honey

Preparation:

1. Divide peaches in half and eliminate pits.

2. Brush cut side of peaches with olive oil.

3. Put on parchment-lined pan and place on 4-inch rack. Cook in NuWave Oven on High power (350°C) for 5-6 mins or until peaches are golden brown and caramelized.

4. Drizzle with honey and serve.

Nutritional Info:

Calories: 61

Fat: 3g

Protein: 1g

Carbs: 10g

Dehydrated cinnamon apple chips

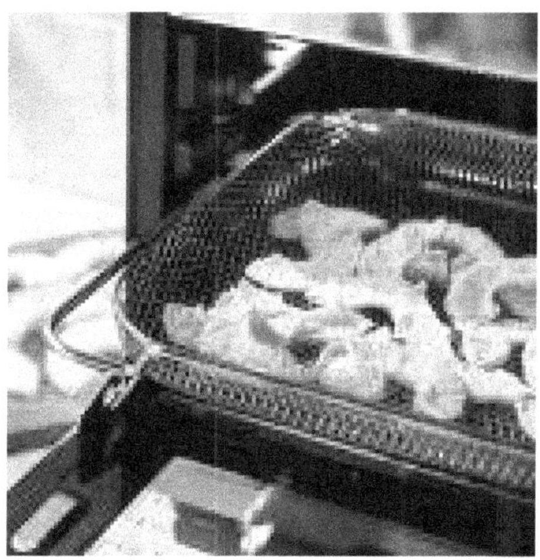

Prep time: 5 mins

Servings: 4

Ingredients:

- 4 large apples

- 1 tbsp. sugar

- 1 tbsp. cinnamon

Preparation:

1. Slice off top side (stem) of apples and then slice apples into rounds around 1/8-inch to ¼-inch thick. This is easiest with a mandolin slicer but can also be done with a sharp knife.

2. Place apple slices in a medium bowl and dash with cinnamon and sugar. Mix gently to coat.

3. Spray 4-inch rack with cooking spray. Arrange apple slices on rack. (Note: You can use both racks to increase cooking area.) Prop dome opens using dome holder to allow steam to escape during dehydration.

4. Cook on Power level 3 (150 degrees F) for 4 hours.

5. Remove from NuWave oven immediately. Allow cooling before serving.

Nutritional Info:

Calories: 90

Total fat: 0g

Carbs: 26g

Protein: 0g

Honey cornbread

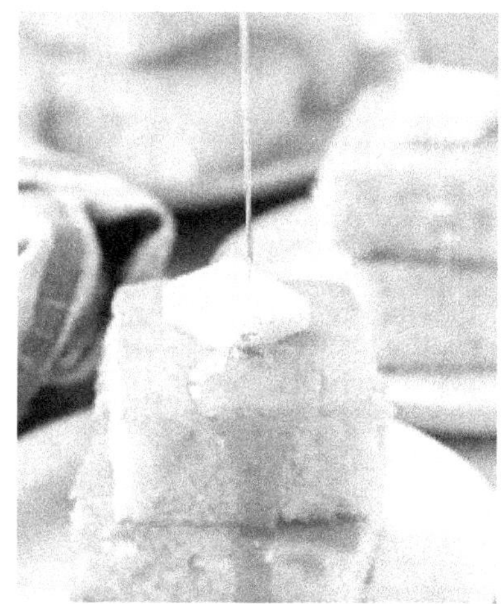

Prep time: 5 mins

Servings: 8

Ingredients:

- 1 c. whole wheat flour

- ¼ c. sugar

- 1 c. heavy cream

- ¼ c. vegetable oil

- 1 c. cornmeal

- ¼ c. honey

- 2 large eggs

- 1 tbsp. baking powder

Preparation:

1. Grease baking pan lightly.

2. In a mixing bowl, mix flour, sugar, cornmeal and baking powder. Add in cream, oil, eggs, and honey. Mix to combine.

3. Pour into baking pan. Bake on 1-inch rack on Power Level High (350 degrees F) for 20 minutes. Let rest for 1-2 minutes before removing from NuWave Oven.

Nutritional Info:

Calories: 170

Total fat: 7g

Carbs: 26g

Protein: 3g

Chocolate zucchini bread

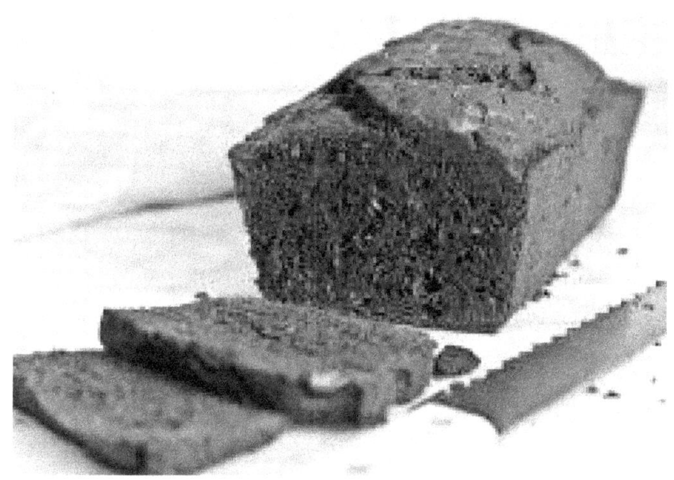

Prep time: 5 mins

Servings: 2

Ingredients:

- 3 medium eggs

- 2 c. sugar

- 1 c. vegetable oil

- 2 c. grated zucchini

- 1 tsp. vanilla extract

- ¾ c. semisweet chocolate chips

- 1/3 c. cocoa powder

- 2 c. wheat flour

- 1 tsp. baking soda

- 1 tsp. sea salt

- 1 tsp. ground cinnamon

Preparation:

1. Spray two baking pans with cooking spray.

2. In a medium mixing bowl, add, cocoa powder, eggs, oil, grated zucchini, vanilla and sugar.

3. Beat well. Fold in flour, baking soda, salt, and cinnamon.

4. Fold in chocolate chips.

5. Pour batter into baking pans. Bake on 1-inch rack on power level High (350°C) for 40-45 mins until knife inserted in centre comes out clear. Allow bread to rest inside the dome for 1-2 minutes before removing from NuWave Oven. Allow cooling before slicing.

Nutritional Info:

Calories: 217.0

Total Fat: 8.0g

Total carbs: 37.0g

Protein: 3.0g

Pineapple banana nut bread

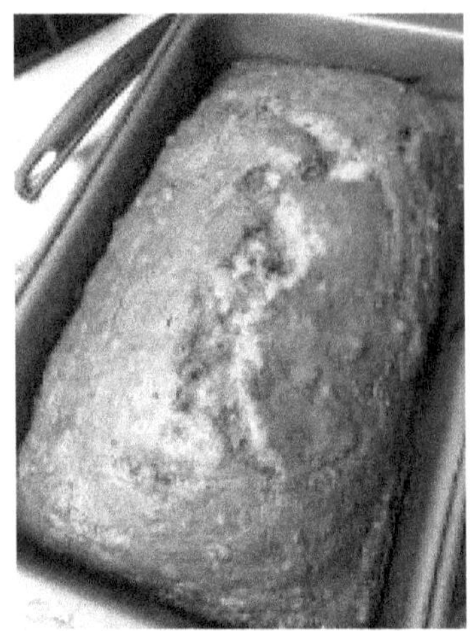

Prep time: 5mins

Servings: 2

Ingredients:

- 3 c. wheat flour

- 1 c. vegetable oil

- ¾ tsp. sea salt

- 1 tsp. baking soda

- 8 oz. crushed pineapple

- 2 c. sugar

- 1 tsp. cinnamon

- 1 c. walnuts

- 3 medium eggs

- 4 ripe bananas

- 2 tsps. vanilla extract

Preparation:

1. Spray baking pans with cooking spray.

2. In a mixing bowl, add sugar, flour, baking soda, salt and cinnamon.

3. Add in walnuts, oil, banana, pineapple, eggs and vanilla. Mix till blended. Pour batter to the pans.

4. Place pans on a 1-inch rack and bakes on High power (350°C) for 45-50 mins or until a toothpick inserted in centre come out clear. Allow rest under the dome for 1-2 minutes before removing from NuWave Oven. Cool before slicing.

Nutritional Info:

Calories: 216

Fat: 10g

Carbohydrate: 30g

Protein: 3g

Blueberry lemon pound cake

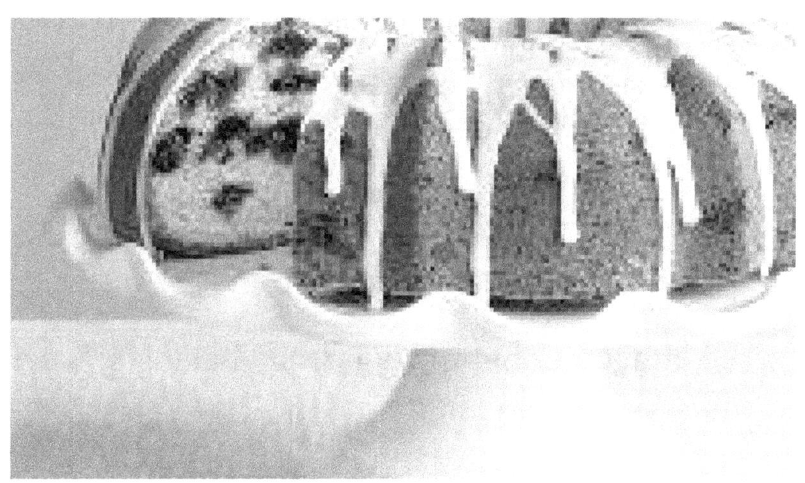

Prep time: 5 mins

Servings: 1

Ingredients:

- 1 tsp. baking powder

- 2 butter sticks

- 1 c. sugar

- ¼ c. fresh lemon juice

- 2 tbsps. lemon zest

- 1 tsp. vanilla extract

- 1/8 tsp. salt

- 4 large eggs

- 2 c. wheat flour

- 1½ c. fresh blueberries

Preparation:

1. Spray the pan with cooking spray.

2. Beat together butter, sugar, and baking powder until smooth and fluffy.

3. Add lemon juice, lemon zest, vanilla, and salt.

4. Mix till combined.

5. Add eggs, one at a time, beating until smooth after each. Add flour and mix until just combined. Fold in blueberries.

6. Spread the batter into the pan. Shake pan to even out the batter.

7. Place Extender Ring on base. Place pan on a 1-inch rack and cook on Power Level 9 (325 degrees F) for 45-50 mins or until knife inserted in centre comes out clear.

8. Remove from NuWave Oven and allow cooling before slicing.

Nutritional Info:

Calories: 265.0

Total Fat: 4.1g

Total carbs: 52.2g

Cranberry bars

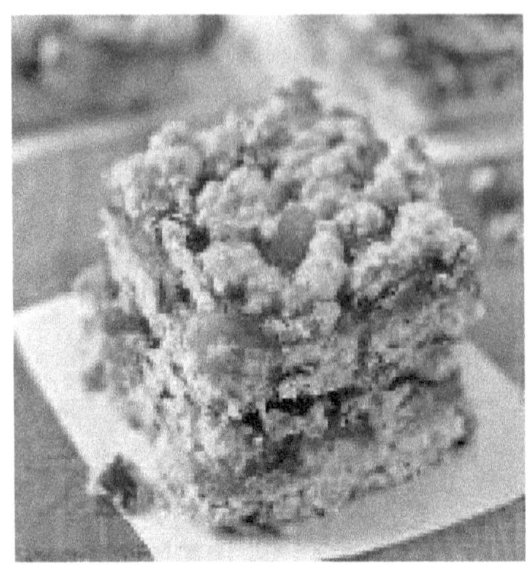

Prep time: 5 mins

Servings: 12

Ingredients:

- 1 ½ c. whole cranberries

- ¾ c. white sugar

- ¾ c. water

- 1 package yellow cake mix

- 6 tbsps. melted butter

- 2 eggs

- ¾ c. rolled oats

- 1 tsp. ground ginger

- 1 tsp. ground cinnamon

- ½ c. brown sugar

Preparation:

1. Spray baking pan with cooking spray.

2. Add cranberries, sugar, and water to saucepan. Cook over medium heat, stirring continuously, until all cranberries pop and mixture thickened for (10-15 mins).

3. Remove from heat and allow cooling.

4. In a mixing bowl, add cake mix, butter, brown sugar, oats, ginger, eggs and cinnamon. Spread 2/3 of the mixture into baking pan. Use back of a spoon to press down evenly to form a crust. Spread cranberry mixture evenly over crust. Top with remaining mixture.

5. Place on 1-inch rack and bake on power level High (350 °C) for 30-35 mins, until top is lightly browned. Allow cooling before cutting.

Nutritional Info:

Calories: 280

Total Fat: 14g

Carbs: 38g

Protein: 3g

Conclusion

Looking at these recipes, it is evident that Nuwave oven is quite a resourceful kitchen equipment and can help in preparing a wide range of delicious meals, be it breakfast, meat, vegetables, seafood, poultry, desserts among many other recipes.

The great feature about using Nuwave oven over other ovens is because of its revolutionary 3 heat technology. It enhances faster operations and minimizes the usage of extra fats to your meals while their nutritional value is retained.

All the recipes in this cookbook are flexible as they do not require a lot of prep work, the ingredients used are easily available locally. The preparation steps are easy to follow as simple terms are used.

In conclusion, it is evident that the nuwave oven is not just a normal piece of kitchen appliance that will stay unused, but it is a portable kitchen equipment that offers great value and service in our world today, that requires easy to prepare the type of foods and at the same time healthy. Nuwave fulfils all this.

Judy Preston

9 781718 785281